Professional Praise for Dr. Friedman and Newman Springs Dental Care

"I have been in dentistry myself for over 30 years and have worked in many offices, and I have to say that Newman Springs Dental Care raises the bar for not only clinical excellence but patient care as well. Every member of the Newman Springs Dental Care team is there because they love the office and the patients. I can honestly say that Dr. Friedman wholeheartedly cares for each and every one of his patients. Not only their dental needs, but he also takes personal interest in them. He and the team continually strive to improve the practice for the patients. I have never seen such dedication to a practice in my career, and the reason for that is because everyone there really cares about their patients and each other. If you want your dental care done right the first time in the most comfortable manner, then please go see Dr. Mitchel Friedman. He and his experienced staff will exceed your expectations!"

Dr. Kelly Bridenstine
Owner of Perfect Smiles Dental, Lenexa, Kansas

"This is an amazing practice. As a practicing dentist, I can assure anyone that they will be well cared for. My team and I have learned much from Dr. Friedman. He is a caring person dedicated to making his patients feel comfortable."

Dr. John Meis
Siouxland Dental, Sioux City, Iowa

"I highly recommend Dr. Friedman to anyone in the Lincroft, New Jersey, area who is looking for quality dentistry. He provides the very best in sedation dentistry and does so with compassion and kindness. By staying up to date with the latest technology, Dr. Friedman ensures that his patients receive the very best care possible. If you're one of the many Americans who has avoided dentistry out of fear or anxiety, Newman Springs Dental Care is the best solution. As a dentist myself, I would choose Dr. Friedman as my dentist if I lived in the Lincroft area."

Dr. David Ahearn
Westport Perfect Smiles, Westport, MA
Owner, Design Ergonomics

"Dr. Friedman is not only a great dentist but also a great person. I know few dentists who are as dedicated, conscientious, and caring as Dr. Friedman. For that reason, I would recommend him to any patient without hesitation. He is truly a leader in his field, highly respected by DENTISTS and his patients."

Dr. Charles Tozzer
Tozzer Dental, Irvine, California
Founder, Dental Care for Children
Instructor, Dental Anesthesia Department, University of Southern California

"If you're looking for the very best in dental care, Dr. Friedman in Lincroft, NJ, is the dentist to provide it. He's a leader in his field and really cares about his patients."

Dr. Tom Peltzer
Central Connecticut Sedation & Sleep Dentist, Plainville, CT

"Dr. Mitchel Friedman is one of America's most prominent sedation dentists and is a leader in providing advanced dental care in a caring environment."

Dr. Gary Cameron
Asheboro Dental Care, Asheboro, NC

"Dr. Mitchel Friedman is one of America's best dentists. He has built an incredible practice and team and is a credit to both his community and the dental profession. We work with dentists all across the country, and I can say Dr. Mitch is truly unique. He offers an impressive array of services to benefit his patients, and for years has been committed to continuous improvement. As a result of these efforts, he now has a very successful practice. His insights to team development, practice growth, and all that comes with running a successful business are incredibly valuable. I am blessed to know and work with Dr. Mitchel Friedman."

Wendy Briggs, RDH
President, The Team Training Institute
Founder, Hygiene Diamonds

Changing Lives
One Smile at a Time

Mitchel Friedman, DDS, MAGD, FDOCS

To my wife Adrienne, who continues to inspire and encourage me every day.

To my children, Gillian, Jared, and Hannah, I am excited to see you making your own paths in life. I have no doubt that you will make the world a better place.

To everyone at Newman Springs Dental Care, let us strive to develop a legacy that continues for generations.

Contents

Foreword

"There has to be a better way!"

I heard these words come from an exasperated dentist nearly 15 years ago. The dentist was unsatisfied with the status quo of the dental patient experience. Too often patients did not get the care they needed because of the obstacles that dental practices put in front of them. He was frustrated by the lack of genuine care and compassion that is still to this day prevalent in dentistry.

The norm was dentists did not address the anxiety that many, maybe most, patients feel about dental procedures. He knew that people were living with dental conditions that were destroying their confidence and quality of life not because they chose to, but because the dental profession simply didn't have or didn't use the techniques and processes that were developing.

That exasperated dentist was Dr. Mitchel Friedman. Unlike many others, he was committed to finding that better way. He took countless hours of courses on the most cutting-edge techniques and technologies to make the dental experience better. He built a team of superstar team members who helped him innovate the patient experience so that even the most anxious people and those with the most severe dental problems could have their lives transformed.

Dr. Friedman has been generous to our profession by teaching many dentists, including me, how to implement his better way.

This book chronicles the wisdom of many years of seeking knowledge, experience, and true compassion for his patients. He has truly found a better way.

John Meis, DDS
CEO, Smart Choice Dentistry and CEO, The Team Training Institute
A proud colleague of Dr. Friedman

Introduction

I wrote this book for you.

This book is for anyone who may have dental anxiety for any reason. This includes tens of millions of people across the United States. Conservatively, this includes hundreds of people in Lincroft and thousands in the surrounding communities.

I wrote it for young adults who are on their own for the first time and looking for a dental home. I wrote it for parents who may be looking for a family dentist. I wrote it for older adults, whose own children are grown and who haven't been to the dentist in years ... or maybe decades because they took care of their family first and neglected themselves.

This book is for anyone who is afraid of the dentist, anyone who cares about someone who has dental anxiety, and anyone who may develop dental anxiety in the future.

It's easy to say that you shouldn't be afraid to go to the dentist. In reality, overcoming dental anxiety can be difficult — but it is possible. I know because I've seen it happen time and time again at our practice.

I want to show you and your loved ones that you can feel comfortable visiting the dentist as part of your normal hygiene routine for decades to come.

Who Am I?

I am a New Jersey boy, born and raised. I graduated from Middletown High School in 1976. Then I enrolled at Rutgers, where I earned my bachelor's degree. I was accepted into the Medical College of Virginia School of Dentistry. I graduated in the top 15 percent of my class and received my doctor of dental surgery in 1984. I returned home to Monmouth County and completed a general practice residency at Monmouth Medical Center.

My education didn't stop after I went into private practice, however. I have completed more than 1,500 hours of continuing education. In 2010, I earned Mastership status in the Academy of General Dentistry. I'll admit that I am proud of this accomplishment, since only 2 percent of dentists earn this distinction.

More important than my mastership, however, are the things I've learned along the way. That includes the many courses I completed on all aspects of dentistry. It also includes the lessons I've learned from my patients. As valuable as coursework can be, experience remains the best teacher. With decades of experience under my belt, I've helped patients with every dental problem you can imagine, which includes working with numerous patients who were fearful about dental care the first time they visited my office.

In addition to my private practice, I serve as a part-time clinical instructor at Monmouth Medical Center, where I teach dental graduates advanced techniques and sedation.

Why I Wrote a Book

Before I started dental school and in the decades since I graduated, I've always wanted to help people.

In all those years, one thing has remained constant. People have always wanted to improve their oral health. The particular problems may vary from patient to patient, but everyone would like to have an attractive, healthy, pain-free smile.

The good news is that no matter what your mouth looks like today, you can be hopeful. The advances in modern dentistry make it possible to repair and replace teeth. We can even fully redesign your smile to bring back your ability to bite and chew, while giving you a new reason to smile.

In this book, you will learn about me and my services. But I want to stress a few things:

- You will not be judged at my office no matter what issues are affecting your smile.
- My goal is to help every patient find a solution to the oral health problems they are facing.
- I also want you to understand that my approach to patient care is based on making you feel as relaxed and comfortable as can be.

As you continue reading, I want you to know that my team and I will be here for you and the people you love most.

1

It's OK If You Haven't Seen a Dentist in Years

More than a decade ago, a young woman came to my office. She had by her own admission avoided going to the dentist for *25 years*. She also knew that something needed to change.

As much as she understood that she needed to make a dental appointment, she was "terrified" about it. As she researched dentists online, she found my practice. After learning a little about us, she decided to call my office. Knowing she could take advantage of our dental sedation helped her feel more comfortable making that first appointment.

By her own description, coming back to the dentist turned out to be easier than she expected. And I'm happy to say that her mouth is still healthy, and she visits my practice regularly for routine cleanings and exams.

She is one of the countless people with dental anxiety we have been able to help at Newman Springs Dental Care over more than 30 years of serving Lincroft and the surrounding area. Seeing the difference that dental care has made in her life and the lives of so many more patients keeps me inspired.

If you can relate to her story, I want to help you, too.

How Common Is Dental Anxiety?

The American Association of Endodontists conducted a survey a few years ago, and they found that 80 percent of people experience some level of dental anxiety. This includes an estimated 5 to 10 percent of respondents who are considered dental phobics, avoiding dental care at all costs.

I'll be honest, 80 percent seems a little high to me, but the statistic may include anyone with even the mildest anxiety. Even using more conservative figures, experts who have studied this for years estimate that between 9 and 20 percent of the U.S. population suffer from dental fear or anxiety. Even with the lower estimates, that's still tens of millions of people in the United States who will go to the dentist only in an absolute dental emergency.

Coincidentally, putting off preventive dental care increases the risk that you will need emergency dental care. And if you are already fearful about going to the dentist, an emergency is hardly an ideal situation for easing your way back into a dental chair.

I can't list every possible reason people may be skittish about going to the dentist, but I can share some of the most common things I have heard from my patients over the last 30 years.

Understandably, many patients are hesitant to make dental appointments because of bad experiences when they were younger. I've heard many such stories from patients. They had dentists who were very critical of even the most minor problems. Some dentists even yelled at them or made them feel ashamed about the condition of their teeth. I wouldn't want to go back to a dentist like that either.

These bad experiences can linger with people for decades. I've treated patients in their 70s and 80s who avoided dental care for decades because of something that happened during their childhood or teenage years.

I've also talked to more people than I could count who said they were afraid to visit the dentist because they were embarrassed about their teeth. The longer this persists, the worse their problems become, and the more embarrassed they feel. As a result, they avoid going to the place where people have the training and skills to help them improve their smiles. And the longer they stay away from the dentist, the harder it is for them to make an appointment.

I also frequently hear from patients who dread going to the dentist because they are convinced it is going to be painful. This could be related to a direct personal experience they had in their youth. This could be because of something they saw in a movie or television show or a story they heard about someone else's bad dental experience. If I thought I was going to get hurt by going somewhere, I would be inclined to avoid visiting that place as well.

Many patients also worry that they may lose control while they are at the dentist's office. An example could be a physical reaction, such as gagging. Maybe they are worried about nervous sweating and uncontrollable squirming in the dental chair. People who are afraid of needles or the drill may be worried about how they might react to seeing or hearing those particular tools.

If one or more of the issues I mentioned — or something I have not mentioned at all — makes you apprehensive about scheduling a trip to the dentist, it's OK. *You* are OK. There's nothing wrong with you.

It's also just as important to know that *you can overcome your anxiety* and learn to manage your fears. I know this because I see it happen every day in my office. I have patients, like the woman I mentioned earlier, who used to live in terror at the thought of a dental cleaning but today visit my team two or more times per year to keep their smiles healthy and looking their best.

How is that possible?

It starts with our approach to our patients. One of our core values (which I'll discuss in greater detail in the next chapter) is that our guests' needs always come first. We want you to feel good about being in our office, and we want you to feel good about who you are. We are going to support you in your journey to a better, healthier smile.

We also offer three levels of dental sedation. I have training in nitrous oxide, oral sedation, and IV sedation. I'll give more details about each form of sedation in chapter 3. The main thing to keep in mind is that we can help you stay relaxed and pain-free no matter what dental treatment you need and regardless of your mild, moderate, or severe anxiety.

We offer a wide range of general, cosmetic, and restorative services as well. If you are unhappy with your teeth for any reason, I have the experience, services, and training to give you a smile you will be happy to share anytime and anywhere.

And last but not least, we work hard to create a welcoming and supportive atmosphere by building close relationships with our patients. You are never "just a mouth" or "just a number" at Newman Springs Dental Care. Every patient is an individual with her or his own reasons for visiting us. We take time to listen to you so we can make dental care easier for you, and so you will keep coming back to see us.

We want to do our part to keep you smiling for years and decades to come through routine, preventive care.

Patient Perspective: Lisa

"I was very apprehensive before I came here — and that's me being complimentary to myself — apprehensive, because really, I was extremely scared," Lisa said. "I was very nervous. I was on the verge of shaking."

At Newman Springs Dental Care, however, she said that she was greeted with smiles and kindness. She even recalled that during her first appointment, Roxanne (one of our dental assistants) took Lisa by the hand and stood by her the whole time she was in the chair.

"Dr. Friedman was very kind as well. He talked to me before to make sure that I was going to be comforted and treated with nothing but sweetness," Lisa said. "He answered all my questions beforehand, and then Miss Pauline came in. And she made me feel like a completely new person.

"I feel healthier walking out the door than I have felt in years, and it was the best experience. I would never be scared to go to a dentist again."

2

Giving Back to Our Community

It would be quite easy to perform dental care without compassion or concern. I know because many patients have told me that's exactly what they experienced at other offices. It's also why it remains so important to me that our patients know we care about them and their health.

This is also why I want to share something with you, something that guides every decision we make at Newman Springs Dental Care. They are our core values:

😊 **Our guests' needs always come first.**

First and foremost, everyone who comes to our office should feel like they are visiting family or friends. We want you to feel good about being here, and we want you to feel good about yourself.

You deserve to be treated with respect and concern, whether you are here as a patient, a parent, or a friend supporting someone else who is anxious about their own appointment. We also know that if you could be anywhere in the world, the dentist's office probably is not the first place on your list. You would rather spend your time with your family and friends, or maybe you would rather be alone curled up with a good book. We know your time is valuable, and we make every effort to stay on schedule so every minute you are with us is worthwhile.

We also understand that dental care can bring with it financial concerns for many people. This is why we provide a range of payment options. We will work with you to find the one that will work best for you and your budget. It's also why we created our own in-house care plan, which many patients prefer to the hassles that can be associated with dental insurance.

Different dental insurance companies have different policies, and even if you have insurance through your work, you may not always know what is covered and what isn't. Dental care shouldn't be about phone calls, paperwork, and fine print. It should be about helping patients.

We created our in-house plan at Newman Springs Dental Care because we wanted to make preventive care simple and affordable for every family in and around Lincroft. When you sign up for our plan, you are dealing with us — the same people you trust and count on to provide your dental care.

Your comfort in our office is essential — physically and mentally. If you are cold, we'll offer you a blanket. If you would like something to drink, let us know. Our comfort menu also includes a number of items to make your dental care less stressful. We have sunglasses to protect your eyes from the overhead lights as well as splatter. We have noise-canceling headphones you can wear if you don't want to listen to the sounds of dental care. You can listen to music or watch something with our Verizon Fios service with more than 1,000 television and music channels.

If you are feeling anxious, we can discuss what we could do differently, or we can help you find a sedation option that will make your visit easier to handle.

If you have questions, we'll be here to answer them before your appointment, in the middle of your treatment, or after you get home and think of something you forgot. We want you to have the information you need to understand your oral health and how to maintain it.

Each and every time you visit, you deserve more than just advanced dentistry. You also deserve to be treated with compassion. You deserve a consistent experience as well. You should know what to expect every time you make an appointment. This starts with compassionate care and courteous treatment along with professional, top-quality service. This helps us build trust with you. I've found that when patients know what to expect, they have an easier time scheduling their next appointment.

☺ Charity and gratitude are part of what we do.

In 2006, my team and I became the first practice in New Jersey to participate in a charity event called **Dentistry From The Heart**. I don't mind saying that we were a bit anxious ourselves that day. We didn't know if anyone would come or what to expect from the day.

What happened turned out to be amazing.

Starting at 7 a.m. that day, our team along with volunteers from other dental offices in the area provided free dental services for 165 patients. These were all individuals who did not have the resources to receive dental care, and this was a way we could help them start getting their oral health back on track.

Since our first year participating in this life-changing event, we have helped more than 1,100 patients receive more than $500,000 in free dental services. Again, this was a cooperative effort by our dentist office and volunteers from other practices, some of whom have started hosting their own events, where my team and I volunteer as well.

I can't take credit for starting this program. That goes to a dentist from Florida, Dr. Vincent Monticciolo, who had become concerned about the residents in his area going without dental care. On Valentine's Day in 2001, he hosted the first event, and he inspired dentists across the country to follow.

I can say that every year we have participated, it has been an uplifting and inspiring experience for me. The generosity and gratitude I get to witness and participate in firsthand is something that carries over into the everyday service we strive to provide for every patient.

9

Dentistry From The Heart has become something we look forward to once a year, but it's only one of the ways we try to give back to our community.

We also participate in **Smiles For Life**. We set aside time each year to give our patients a chance to help themselves while helping children as well. During this event, patients can sign up for professional teeth whitening. All of the proceeds go to charity — half is shared with local organizations and half goes to the Smiles For Life Foundation. The foundation supports children's charities all across North America, including the Ronald McDonald House, St. Jude's Children's Research Hospital, Feed the Children, and more.

Locally, we have used proceeds from our teeth whitening event to support **Parker Family Health Center** in Red Bank. The center's mission is to provide free care for Monmouth County residents who don't have insurance or other means to pay for medical treatment.

At Halloween, we host a **Candy Buy Back** program as well. It's a win-win-win situation. Kids gets some money. You have less candy at your house (so less temptation to eat cavity-causing sweets). And all the candy we collect is shipped overseas to men and women serving our country in the military. It's our way of showing them some appreciation for the sacrifices they are making for all of us.

Locally, we are honored to award three **$500 scholarships** annually for area high school seniors who are planning to enter careers in dentistry, medicine, or another area of health care. These awards have been presented to one graduate each from Holmdel High School, Middletown High School North, and Middletown High School South every year since 2010.

😊 We aim to be hyper-convenient and service oriented.

What does "hyper-convenient" mean? We do like our office location, but that's not what I'm referring to here. For us, hyper-convenient means being available at times that work with our patients' schedules. Many people can't take time off work to schedule dental visits, and many parents don't like the idea of taking their kids out of school for cleanings and exams. This is why we have evening office hours twice a week, early morning hours once per week, and Saturday hours twice every month.

We also offer same-day appointments, especially for patients dealing with dental emergencies. Call us in the morning, and we'll set aside time to see you that day. We also use advanced technology to complete your treatment in a single visit whenever possible. For broken, cracked, and damaged teeth, we can design and place your dental crown while you wait with our CEREC technology and in-office crown milling machine.

☺ Excellence is achieved through accountability and thoroughness.

Earlier I noted that our goal is for every patient to have consistently good experiences during each visit with us. This is why my team uses accountability forms. This keeps us alert to our patients' needs ... and it serves as a reminder to live up to the standards we set for ourselves.

We know we aren't perfect, although we strive to do our best for every patient and for each other every day. It's why every member of my team is open to learning how to improve and teaching each other new and better ways to serve our patients.

You know from your daily life and your career that technology is constantly changing. I am constantly reading and learning about these advances to find equipment and technology that make your dental care pain-free and stress-free.

Accountability is a means of providing positive reinforcement to one another, as well. That's one of the reasons we play what we call the "Caught Ya Card" game. Each day, our team members identify another teammate who went the extra mile to help a patient or another member of our team as a way of bolstering the values we strive to uphold. We even award prizes for this every four weeks.

I also believe that my team can help every patient. This belief guides how we treat everyone who sits in one of our dentist chairs. I also want to be able to communicate with you honestly about your dental situation. The more I can do to help you understand, the more likely you are to make an informed decision about your oral health.

🙂 **We are warm, caring, enthusiastic, and lighthearted, and we treat patients like family.**

Our concern for you doesn't stop when you walk in the office and end when you walk out the door. We want to help you celebrate your successes and special occasions.

We build personal relationships with our patients. We *want* to celebrate your birthdays along with our own. We have sent cards to encourage our patients who are sick or going through hard times. We also send thank you cards to show our patients our gratitude for the things they do for us. If you happen to have a dental appointment on a holiday, don't be surprised if you see us dressed up to get in the spirit.

As part of this effort to keep our atmosphere fun and relaxed, we are happy to put on a TV show or video for you to watch during your service. It you'd like a warm towel or a cup of coffee, we're happy to offer them. When you go home, we'll send you off with a goodie bag.

If you use social media, we invite you to like us on Facebook. We love interacting with our patients online, and who knows, you might have a chance to win one of our contests while you're at it. In fact, we hope you will check in on Facebook with our free Wi-Fi during your visit.

We won't forget about you, either. If you have a treatment that calls for multiple visits, we'll stay in contact to keep you and your oral health on the right track.

Now that you've learned about the things that are important to us, I hope you have a better understanding of who I am. It's important to me to get to know you and how I can make general dentistry better for you and the people you love.

Our Mission

To me, our work with Dentistry From The Heart is a reflection of the mission, culture, and values that I want to promote at my practice. You should know what to expect from us, which is why I'm sharing our mission statement here:

Newman Springs Dental Care is a team of professionals dedicated to helping our patients achieve and maintain their optimal dental health.

Always striving to exceed our patients' expectations, we will treat them with honesty, care, respect, and comfort.

The team is committed to continuing education, constant never-ending improvement, and excellence. In this pursuit, we are unwilling to compromise our values.

Through the sharing of this mission, we will enhance the lives of our patients.

Any business, church, or civic organization can have a mission statement. It only matters if the people involved actively work to live up to that mission. I'm proud to say that this is something my team and I strive to uphold for every patient, every day.

Patient Perspective: Kathleen

"I've been afraid of the dentist my whole life. I've had some negative experiences," Kathleen said. After finding our practice online, she decided to give professional dental care another try. "It was the most wonderful experience I could imagine. Everything about it, from the way your staff treated me — everybody, from the beginning, they were encouraging. They were passionate. They were friendly. The procedures went well. I don't remember much of them — and that was a good thing. It took me a little while to wake up, but I was fine after that."

It's also why she has returned to our office multiple times, even though she was afraid before her first visit.

"I knew I needed to do it, but I didn't have the courage to do it because I had extreme anxiety," Kathleen said. "I'd had the swallowing reflex problem. My blood pressure went sky high."

After learning more about Newman Springs Dental Care and talking to me, she felt that all her concerns would be handled.

"So I was relaxed. I was relaxed coming up here. I was relaxed when I woke up," Kathleen said. "And I was not afraid to come again."

3

Sedation Dentistry

In 2001, I came to a realization. Something had to change.

At the time, I believed I had been doing a good job explaining the benefits of preventive dental care, such as a healthy mouth and a beautiful smile. Yet, being able to explain those benefits often was not enough to convince many people to make a dental appointment or to proceed with a treatment they needed.

Dental fear, it seemed, was a huge obstacle for many people. They understood what could happen if they didn't do something. Still, their anxiety stopped them from receiving what would be beneficial care.

I knew that I had to do something that would make it easier for those patients to get the help they needed. This is when I decided to get trained in sedation dentistry.

Since then, I have completed multiple certifications and advanced training in dental sedation. It's the reason I can offer nitrous oxide and oral sedation. It's also why I can offer IV sedation, which few general dentists will provide. As more people have learned about our sedation options, I've found it gratifying to know that countless patients have received the care they needed.

Are *You* a Good Candidate for Sedation?

Dental anxiety affects people from all walks of life — including dental professionals. In fact, a member of our team, Jennifer, describes herself as a "high-fear patient."

Like many people, she had a bad experience. In her case, it was with her pediatric dentist. Although this happened many years ago, she still has difficulty when it's her turn to be a patient.

She no longer needs sedation during her visits, but she understands all the emotions that fearful patients go through when they come to our office. She has shared that knowledge with me and the other members of our team. This has helped us be more understanding when we are assisting anxious patients.

In chapter 1, I described some of the common reasons patients have told me that they feel uncomfortable about visiting any dentist. Let's review some of them because if you share any of these concerns, sedation may be perfect for you.

The single most common reason people are fearful is that, like Jennifer, they had a bad experience when they were younger. I've even had patients in their 70s and 80s who were making their first dental visits since childhood for this very reason.

Pain or fear that their treatment will be painful is another widely stated reason for avoiding dentistry. This may go back to an earlier experience as well.

If this is a concern for you, you owe it to yourself to find a modern dentist who understands how to eliminate pain. That includes giving anesthetic or sedation time to take effect. At our practice, we will make sure you are completely numb before we begin. If you ever feel like you need to take a break during your care, you only need to raise your hand to let us know.

Patients who have sensitive gag reflexes have a very legitimate reason for not wanting to go somewhere where people will be putting hands and tools in their mouths. The American Psychological Association also has reported that anxiety-induced gagging is a real issue. Some people are more likely to gag as a direct result of their dental anxiety. To put this another way, if you already feel anxious about gagging, that anxiety can increase the likelihood that you may gag during your dental visit.

For multitudes of people, embarrassment about their teeth is a source of general anxiety. Once again, this could be directly tied to an experience from their younger days. If anyone has tried to shame you about your smile, then you may worry your dentist might do the same. While it is an understandable concern, it's not something you need to worry about at Newman Springs Dental Care.

Neither I nor anyone on my team will judge you or your smile. In fact, we will do the opposite. We'll make every effort to give you a reason to feel good about your smile again through words of encouragement, some form of cosmetic or restorative treatment, or both.

How Sedation Dentistry Can Help

I've seen how sedation has allowed patients to manage all the concerns and fears I've mentioned and many others. When patients are sedated, they feel calmer and much more relaxed.

Even if you don't personally experience dental anxiety, you may relate to having anxiety about a test, a first date, or giving a speech in front of an audience. You know how that affects you mentally, but it can have physical effects as well. As Kathleen mentioned in her testimonial, her blood pressure would rise as a result of her dental anxiety.

Many people respond to anxiety by producing cortisol, a hormone associated with stress and "fight-or-flight" feelings. When you remain stressed for extended periods of time, it can increase your anxious feelings. It also can contribute to digestive issues, headaches, memory issues, and weight gain. I certainly don't want you to feel stressed about being in one of our chairs.

I've also had patients tell me that they have trouble sleeping the night before a dental appointment. Sleep problems can be a consequence of anxiety.

Sedation will put your mind at ease. By receiving this medication, your anxiety and stress will fade away. For some patients, just knowing sedation will be part of their visit helps them get a good night's rest before they see us.

Sedation also is proven to block pain. In fact, that's a big part of the reason sedation has been used in dental and medical care for more than a century.

Back in 1772, just a few years before the United States won our independence from England, chemist Joseph Priestley isolated nitrous oxide. This also came to be known as "laughing gas" because of the euphoric feelings many people described after inhaling it.

A few years later, Horace Wells, an American dentist, witnessed a public demonstration involving nitrous oxide. During the demonstration, a man who had been breathing laughing gas bumped his leg, but the man could not recall doing so after the gas was removed. This gave Wells an idea. Using himself as a test subject, he instructed an assistant to pull one of his teeth while he was under the effects of nitrous oxide. Convinced of the benefits, he started using nitrous oxide as a normal part of his dental practice, performing painless dental procedures.

In time, more people learned of the pain-blocking benefits of laughing gas, and the equipment for delivering the gas improved, giving the dentist greater control. Today, many dentists and physicians use it as a normal part of their care.

While some practices only offer nitrous oxide, it's just one of the sedation options I can offer you. I'll have more to say about laughing gas and my other sedation options in the next chapter. In the meantime, I want to continue discussing ways sedation could help you or someone you love.

Just as sedation can dull your response to pain, it can reduce the sensations that could trigger a gag reflex. This too can reduce anxiety-related gagging. In both cases, this can make it easier for you to complete a cleaning or other dental treatment.

I want to close by reminding you of a quote from my patient Kathleen at the end of the previous chapter. Referring to her treatments, she said, "I don't remember much of them — and that was a good thing." For her and many anxious patients, being able to get dental care without any memory of what happens is the best of both worlds.

This makes it much easier for anyone to get through more complicated procedures, such as full-mouth reconstruction. Sedation can keep you still and relaxed, which makes any treatment less difficult for me and my assistants. For you, the patient, it may feel like you just took a long nap.

As you can see, there are many benefits to sedation dentistry. Next, I'll give some information that could help you determine which sedation option is best for you.

Patient Perspective: Jim

Jim first visited us, in his own words, after "years of neglect and lack of follow-through with dental procedures." After talking with me, he appreciated that I was professional and nonjudgmental in discussing the procedure he would need.

"The sedation was good for me because I had a lot of work to get done. I had some poor experiences in the past, and the experience was fantastic," Jim said. "Not only was the staff professional, Mitch was a lot of fun. The staff was a lot of fun. We had some laughs along the way."

And as a result of his care, Jim feels much better about his teeth.

"I'm much more comfortable laughing, smiling now based on the results, and I'd have to recommend this to anybody who's been in this position of — particularly like mine, who spent some time away from the dentist and away from doing what they need to do," he said.

Jim liked that he knew what was going to happen, and he knew what the final results would be.

"I couldn't be happier."

4

Your Comfort Is Always the Priority

In 2001, I decided to get the necessary training so I could offer sedation dentistry. I saw a need for this service in Lincroft and our neighboring communities.

There was one problem. At that time, New Jersey did not offer sedation training for general dentists like me. As a lifelong learner, I was determined to get the education I needed. I took additional courses and hands-on training to ensure my patients' comfort and safety.

When the New Jersey State Board of Dentistry created a permit program in 2004, I enrolled immediately. I was one of the first dentists in the Garden State to receive a permit to offer oral sedation.

Not long after that, I also met the Fellowship requirements for the Dental Organization for Conscious Sedation. To meet these standards, I had to complete at least 75 hours of continuing education and have at least 50 documented sedation cases. I exceeded those standards, and I kept learning so I could offer more sedation options for my patients.

In 2009, I completed an 80-hour course offered at the oral surgery and anesthesia departments at St. Joseph's Medical Center in Paterson, NJ. With this training, I became, and remain, one of the few general dentists in New Jersey who is licensed to provide IV sedation at my practice.

My team and I make a conscientious effort to exceed all state and national safety requirements so we can continue to offer three forms of sedation at our practice. Every member of my team has been certified in Healthcare Provider CPR by the American Heart Association.

We now perform more than 400 sedation procedures every year, so it would be fair to say that at Newman Springs Dental Care, sedation dentistry is an everyday service.

Different Kinds of Dental Sedation

Many dentists offer nitrous oxide, but few have completed the extensive training required to offer multiple levels of sedation.

I agree that mild sedation is great for many patients, but I want to be able to help as many people as I can. When I first decided to get certified to offer dental sedation, I was doing it because I knew there was a need to help patients who had avoided dental care for years. By offering a range of options, I am able to assist patients with even severe anxiety to get the dental care they needed.

With this in mind, here's what you can expect from each kind of sedation.

Nitrous oxide is the mildest form of sedation I use in my practice. One of its biggest benefits is that it takes effect and wears off within minutes. All you have to do is breathe.

Using a nasal mask, we can deliver a combination of nitrous oxide and oxygen to you. The nitrous oxide can be adjusted for each individual when it is inhaled. As it takes effect, you will notice a calming, relaxing sensation. You won't feel any pain, and you won't feel like you are going to gag.

You will continue breathing the gas throughout your cleaning or other treatment. When we are finished, we simply turn off the gas, so you can inhale 100 percent oxygen. As you exhale any remaining nitrous oxide, you will return to feeling like you did before you started breathing the gas.

For patients with mild anxiety, nitrous oxide is a simple and effective way to feel at ease throughout their appointments. At the same time, many patients with moderate or severe anxiety will step down to nitrous oxide as they become more comfortable with us.

We've even had some patients who have overcome their anxiety to a point that they no longer need any sedation for routine care.

Oral sedation is a step up from nitrous oxide, and I recommend this to patients with moderate to severe dental anxiety. This is as easy as taking a dose of medication before your appointment. You should be aware that you *must* arrange for someone else to drive you to and from your appointment if you choose oral sedation. This can be a trusted family member, friend, or co-worker.

It will take longer for you to feel the full effects of oral sedation. However, like nitrous oxide, oral sedation will help you feel at ease during your visit with us. Again, you won't feel any pain, and you won't have to worry about gagging. After your treatment is over, you may continue to feel sedated for a few hours. Any time you choose this sedation option, your driver will take you home so you can rest until the effects wear off.

Oral sedation isn't just for patients who experience dental anxiety. Many patients who have no trouble with a routine cleaning will request oral sedation for something a little more complex, such as a root canal treatment. The medication will keep you calm and pain-free well after the procedure is complete.

IV sedation is the strongest form of sedation that I provide. Even though it is our highest level of sedation, I do have patients with severe anxiety who receive this for all dental care — including cleanings.

When a patient comes to our office, we monitor his or her blood pressure, pulse rate, and blood oxygen level. This helps us know whether the sedation is working and that it is being administered safely and correctly. We want you to feel calm and composed.

As with nitrous oxide, you will feel the effects of IV sedation very quickly. Often, it takes less than a minute. In addition to remaining pain-free, you won't remember your cleaning, root canal, implant placement, or any other dental procedure you receive.

IV sedation does have something in common with oral sedation. If you receive IV sedation, you will need hours for the effects to wear off completely. You also must arrange for someone you trust to take you home to rest after you receive IV sedation.

Other Ways for You to Stay Comfortable

Even if you aren't interested in dental sedation, my team and I are going to make every effort to help you be comfortable any time you visit.

Say you are lying back in a dental chair. A dental professional is standing over you, looking inside your mouth. In this situation, you may find yourself looking into a bright light. This is why we will gladly offer you protective sunglasses to wear during your appointment. We don't want to hurt your eyes while keeping your mouth healthy.

If you live or work with other people, then you are aware that different people can have very different opinions about what is a "comfortable" room temperature. Knowing this, some patients may feel chilly at our office. If you are one of them, just let us know. We have blankets on hand, and we are happy to share them with our guests.

Noise is another problem for a lot of patients. You may not have any issues having your teeth cleaned, but that doesn't mean you want to hear the sounds of dental equipment being moved around and used. If you would rather drown out the sound, we can loan you a pair of our noise-canceling headphones. You can use them to listen to music or while watching one of your favorite television shows. (I do have a word of warning: You may miss one of my great jokes if you have the headphones on.)

Even if you are not interested in sedation, I bet you still don't want to be in pain. This is why we use local anesthetic, and to be more specific, it's why we deliver it in a way that keeps you from feeling even the slightest prick of a syringe.

Using a cotton swab, we apply a small amount of a numbing gel to the area of your mouth where we will be working. Then, we use a tool called The Wand. This is a high-tech, computer-assisted system for delivering pain-preventing medicine. With this tool, we can gently apply pressure where the anesthetic is needed. Then the computer controls the flow of the local anesthetic.

This also helps reduce the spread of the anesthetic to other areas of the mouth, so you don't have that numb-all-over feeling when you are finished. If needed, we will have you rinse your mouth before offering you an analgesic, such as Advil or Tylenol. By taking this before the anesthetic wears off, you will experience less soreness from your procedure.

As a final touch, we will offer you a nice, warm towel if you'd like to freshen up before you head home or back to work.

Before You Decide on a Sedation Option

You are always welcome to ask questions before you schedule an appointment at my office. There is no limit to the number of questions you can ask, and no question is off limits. I'll be happy to answer anything you want to know about sedation dentistry in general or about our sedation and comfort options.

I want you to make the right choice for you. To do that, you deserve all the information you need to make a knowledgeable decision.

Sedation has allowed us to provide preventive, restorative, and cosmetic services for thousands of patients who may not have come to the dentist without it. To me, the biggest benefit of sedation dentistry is giving patients a reason to feel comfortable sitting in a dentist's chair again.

When you are ready to schedule your visit, my team and I look forward to helping you.

Patient Perspective: Terry Ann

Terry Ann will tell you that her teeth were in bad shape when she first came to Newman Springs Dental Care.

"When I first came here, I was expecting to just really find out about getting false teeth because I thought I had reached that point in my life because they were in very, very bad condition," she recalled.

She remembers walking into the office, and she remembers sitting down in one of our chairs for her appointment.

"And I don't remember anything after that," she said with a laugh. "How long it was, I have no perception."

Terry Ann does know that coming to see me has made a difference in her life.

"People will see me, and they can't believe the difference in me. And it's not just my teeth. It's everything about me," she said, adding, "They say, 'You know, you look great. What did you do?'"

Terry Ann tells them that she had her teeth done, and they reply that they think it was something else. At the same time, she did acknowledge that fixing her smile has improved her confidence.

"I think I stand a little taller. I think I walk a little straighter, and it's just really changed how I feel about myself. I'm happier," she said. "When I see who I am in the mirror, it's kind of what I wanted to see."

5

Dental Implants and Other Ways to Restore Your Teeth

Terry Ann's story also serves as a nice introduction to restorative dentistry. Sedation allowed her to restore her smile, and that helped her feel better about herself, too.

She is just one of the countless patients who have had similar experiences at my practice. Like Terry Ann, lots of people are bothered by the condition of their teeth or lack of teeth, since missing teeth are a concern for millions of people across the country.

If you are in this situation, I have two goals in mind when you come to see me. First, I want to restore the full function of your teeth. Your mouth is where you start breaking down your food. If you aren't able to chew well, then you will have a harder time digesting your food and getting the nutrition you need. Second, I want to restore the appearance of your smile.

These are not mutually exclusive goals. You can have teeth replacements that work practically as well as natural teeth, and your replacement teeth can look and feel like real teeth, too.

Dental Implants

Some of you probably know people who have dental implants. Some of you know people who have implants, even if you don't know that they have implants. And some of you are just learning about dental implants.

The first thing you should know is that *dental implants have transformed modern restorative dentistry*. So, what are they, and why should you care?

Implants are prosthetics, much like a prosthetic leg or hand. Dental implants replace the roots of missing teeth. This means even if you have an implant, other people aren't going to see it. Modern implants, also known as root-form implants, have proven to be successful in more than 95 percent of cases. It's also become common for patients to have implants for 40 or 50 years. When someone gets dental implants, they are getting teeth replacements that are stronger, more stable, and more secure than at any other time in human history.

How are implant-supported teeth replacements better than ever? With titanium implants, osseointegration occurs. Through this process, the implants fuse directly with your jawbone. That provides a more stable and secure foundation to support your teeth replacements.

It's also good for the health of your jaw. When the implants are in place, they stimulate your jawbone every time you bite or chew, much like the roots of natural teeth. Your jaw responds to this pressure by creating new bone tissue. This works to prevent the bone loss that occurs when someone loses but does not replace their teeth.

I have used dental implants for patients in a variety of situations. A single implant can be used to replace a missing tooth. Multiple implants can replace multiple teeth, or a series of implants can replace a whole row of teeth. The number of implants will vary depending on how many teeth are missing and where the implants are placed.

To help you understand just how beneficial implants can be, I want to describe how I use them to replace one or both arches of teeth in someone's mouth.

Implant-supported dentures

Implant-supported dentures are anchored to your jawbone, whereas traditional dentures rest on the outside of your gums. This is why traditional dentures frequently slip out of place or come loose. The instability of dentures makes it more difficult to eat as well. Many people will turn to denture adhesive to help hold dentures in place. This may offer some limited benefits, but the adhesive can have a funny taste, which can interfere with the flavor of your food.

In contrast, eating with implant-supported dentures is nearly the same as eating with a full set of teeth. The implants provide a direct connection from your jawbone to your dentures. As a result, people with implants can restore 90 percent or more of the biting power of someone with all their natural teeth. In other words, you can eat what you want, and you won't worry that your replacement teeth will come out.

Implant-supported bridges

Let's say you don't need to replace a complete row of teeth, but you are missing a few teeth in one part of your mouth. A traditional dental bridge might be one way of fixing this. However, we must grind down neighboring teeth to provide support for your bridge. As a dentist, I don't like to remove anything from otherwise healthy teeth, but that's necessary with this kind of bridge.

Traditional bridges will fail sooner or later. Additionally, the dental cement used to bond the bridge to neighboring teeth will wash out, and the teeth supporting your bridge may deteriorate. When one or both of these things happen, the bridge can become loose or damage other teeth.

Dental implants can resolve these issues and keep your bridge secure in your mouth. With implants, your bridge is not bonded to neighboring teeth. It's attached to the implants, which are held in place by your jawbone. I don't have to do anything to your remaining healthy teeth. I simply place your implants, and when your mouth has healed, I customize the bridge to attach them.

Your implant-supported bridge will look like a natural part of your smile, and it will restore the function you lost when your teeth were missing.

Implant-supported crowns

If you are missing a single tooth, the old way of fixing it was grinding down the two nearest teeth and using them to support a dental bridge. This is similar to the process I just described but with a smaller bridge. This also means you would be in a similar situation. Your bridge would be cemented to nearby teeth, and likewise, it would give out in time.

By getting a dental implant and a dental crown, you will be replacing your whole tooth. The implant replaces the missing root, while the dental crown takes the place of the natural crown. Since I don't have to alter any neighboring teeth to complete this procedure, you will have a better chance of keeping those teeth healthy.

My Approach to Implant Placement

I like to stay on the cutting edge of dental technology. For a patient who may be getting a dental implant, the evaluation may start with a 3-D digital scan of his or her mouth. Three-dimensional scans give me a much better idea of whether someone has enough bone to support an implant. The 3-D images also help me plan the implant placement and place each implant precisely so it can provide the most support for your replacement tooth or teeth.

Through a combination of technology, training, and experience, I'm able to place implants and add restorations in a matter of months. I mention this because I've had several patients come to me after they visited other dentists and were told it might take more than a year before they could enjoy the full benefits of their implants.

I don't think you should have to wait that long. It helps that I can handle every step of the process — from the evaluation, to the planning, to the placement, and finally to the restoration — right here in my office. Since I control the procedure from start to finish, I can give you a better idea of how long it will take.

Other Ways to Restore the Function of Your Teeth

Losing a tooth isn't the only reason you may need to repair your smile. If your teeth become broken, cracked, or decayed, then a dental crown could be the perfect solution. An all-ceramic crown can give you back your ability to bite and chew comfortably.

Using 3-D imaging, we design and create a dental crown that restores the shape and appearance of your natural tooth. Since we have a CEREC milling machine in our office, we can design, create, and place your crown in a matter of 60 minutes or less. You won't wait for weeks to get your permanent crown.

Crowns aren't your only option for tooth repairs, either. Depending on how extensive the damage is and how quickly you act to fix your damaged tooth, you may be able to get dental bonding or a dental filling instead. We use tooth-colored fillings at our office to treat tooth decay. This way, you can fix your tooth without other people knowing you ever had a cavity. For small chips and cracks, we can use the same composite resin material for dental bonding. This is a fast, simple, and effective way to build back what was lost in your tooth.

On the other hand, if you wait too long to get a repair, you may need more than a filling or a dental crown. When the decay spreads too deep, it can lead to an infection, which will require a root canal to repair.

I am aware that root canal treatments don't have the best reputation. For some people, they are the exact reason they have dental anxiety. This is unfortunate because your root canal can be easy and pain-free with sedation dentistry. You might not believe that if your impression of root canals comes from movies or from someone who had a root canal decades ago.

In my experience, too often a patient will ignore an infection in hopes that it will get better. It doesn't. When the toothache finally gets to be too much, he or she will come in to get a root canal. The reality is that root canals take away your infection, which in turn takes away pain. Root canals don't cause more pain. And when the procedure is finished, I'll restore the tooth with a dental crown so you can smile and eat like you did before the infection occurred.

Why Restorative Dentistry Is Important to You and Me

Over the past three decades, I've helped thousands of patients with thousands of dental issues. So many patients have come to my office convinced that there is little to no hope of having healthy smiles again. Happily, I can say that those patients have been pleasantly surprised. Countless people have left my office able to eat, smile, and hold their heads high again.

I do take satisfaction in making the physical changes to restore someone's teeth. However, that is nothing compared to the feeling I get when I see someone's renewed sense of self-confidence. The restorative benefits you just read about and cosmetic improvements are an integral part of what I do. My team and I aren't just here to fix your teeth. We also want you to enjoy your life.

Patient Perspective: John M.

John has been a patient at Newman Springs Dental Care for around 25 years. He considers our team to be like family.

"Dr. Friedman, he's become a friend of mine over the years, and I wouldn't go anywhere else," John said.

A few years ago, John needed to have a bridge replaced, and he decided to get dental implants to support his new bridge.

"The implant work he did for me was a piece of cake. I come in, I come out. In less than two hours, the implants were done," John said. "Anybody that needs an implant, I would recommend Dr. Friedman for sure. He's the man."

6

You Deserve to Love Your Smile

Some people are particularly memorable. I recall one patient who had a large and impressive mustache. He also had what he considered bad teeth. I did an exam, and with the help of my team, we were able to fix his teeth so they looked nice.

When he came back for his follow-up appointment, his big, bushy mustache was gone. He'd shaved it off. As it turned out, the main reason he'd grown out his whiskers was to hide his teeth when he smiled or spoke. Now that he liked the look of his teeth, he didn't want to hide his smile anymore.

And I'll never forget a patient who was 80 years old and a widower. He'd lost his wife 10 years earlier, and he finally decided that he would get 11 dental implants (with the help of sedation) to replace his missing teeth.

With his new teeth, he decided to start dating again. I'm also happy to report that the last time I saw him, he was loving life and still grateful to have his smile back.

These are just two of many examples I am happy to share with you. I've observed that how people feel about their teeth can make a huge difference in their quality of life. When people feel embarrassed or ashamed to smile, it has a negative effect on how they interact with other people.

Many patients have come to me after habitually hiding their smiles for years — and most of them didn't grow oversized mustaches. To this day, people come to my office who feel compelled to hide their mouths with their hands any time they speak. They also may use napkins, tissues, books, magazines, or anything else they can find to conceal their smiles. Frequently, these patients will talk as little as possible so as not to reveal their teeth.

I want you to feel confident and comfortable with your smile. I want you to be able to apply for a job, go out on a date, or just enjoy dining out with your friends without feeling self-conscious about taking a bite or telling a joke.

If my three decades of experience have taught me anything, it's that I can help you create a better smile — a smile that you won't want to hide!

Cosmetic Dentistry Can Give You Confidence in Your Smile

Time and time again, I have observed cosmetic dentistry change how patients view themselves. I've seen people smile wide and shed a few happy tears after seeing their new teeth. My team and I always feel good during these moments.

So many more people could benefit from cosmetic improvements to their smiles. And yet, fear of the dentist can prevent someone from doing something that could have a lasting impact on his or her daily life.

Just like the (formerly) mustached patient and the widower, you too can feel good about sharing your smile with the world. No matter what you think of your teeth today, you can have a great smile tomorrow.

If you want to make a change, my team and I can show you how.

Ways You Could Improve Your Smile

What if you have a full set of healthy teeth, but you still don't like how they look? The good news is that there are many ways you can improve your smile. Let's look at some of your options.

Stained teeth are one of the most common cosmetic concerns I hear from my patients. It's a fact of life that our teeth are more likely to look yellower or darker as we get older. Nearly all the foods we eat and the beverages we drink add to the stains on our teeth.

It's also possible that your teeth can become discolored for other reasons. Illnesses and injuries can affect the shade of your smile. Even certain medications can alter the appearance of your teeth.

So what can you do to help your "pearly whites" live up to their nickname again?

Professional teeth whitening is one option. This is a safer and more effective alternative to products you've probably seen in stores and advertised on TV. Professional products can produce results in as little as one visit to our office. These are more potent than commercial products, which is why you should only get them from dental professionals. We first design a custom-made whitening tray for your teeth to apply the gel so that you can have a brighter smile from ear to ear.

After you whiten your teeth, we know that you'll want to keep them healthy and looking great. Our Whitening for Life program is an easy way to do that. For a one-time fee of $99, we will make custom whitening trays for you and give you gel that can make your teeth four to six shades whiter. We'll give you more gel at no additional cost at your routine six-month checkups. A white, bright smile can be your reward for doing what you should to keep your mouth healthy.

As effective as whitening can be on stained teeth, it doesn't work well on other kinds of discoloration. It's so important to talk to a dental professional *before* you use any whitening product.

For patients who need another option for a whiter smile, **dental veneers** are incredibly effective. Dental veneers can be compared to false fingernails. You may have a healthy fingernail, but it may not look as nice as you would like. By getting false nails, your hands can look that much nicer. Similarly, you may have teeth that are perfectly healthy but are just not as white as you would like them to be. By getting veneers bonded to the front of your teeth, you can have a smile that is both healthy *and* attractive.

If you are interested in getting veneers, we can give you an idea of what it will look like before you make your decision. After taking your picture, we can use our Smile-Vision computer program to show you how your teeth could look with veneers. With proper care, your veneers can last for decades, which makes them a better investment than false fingernails.

Veneers also have one advantage over teeth whitening that you may want to consider. Dental veneers are more stain-resistant than teeth. You may be able to maintain your new smile for longer when you have veneers. You still need to brush, floss, and have regular dental cleanings, but you might have an easier time keeping your bright, white smile with veneers.

In addition to having "pearly white" smiles, people also like to have teeth that are straight and evenly spaced. If you have mild spacing issues or your teeth are slightly crooked, veneers may be a good option. This will give you the appearance of a perfectly aligned smile.

If the alignment and spacing problems are bigger than veneers can fix, you can consider orthodontic solutions. Two great options that have helped many of my patients are **Invisalign** and Six Month Smiles. Both are different from traditional braces in their own way, but they have proven to be effective at straightening smiles.

Invisalign uses a series of clear plastic aligners, similar to smaller, transparent mouthguards, to gently push teeth into new positions. Most people won't realize you have them on while you are wearing them. You wear each aligner for a few weeks at a time, then swap it for the next one in the series to keep your teeth moving in the right directions.

Invisalign has been used to close gaps between teeth. It has helped straighten crooked and crowded teeth. It has corrected overbites, underbites, crossbites, and open bites as well. For patients with mild or moderate alignment issues, Invisalign is often a more comfortable and convenient option than traditional metal-and-wire braces.

Six Month Smiles can be used to correct many of the same issues as Invisalign. Like traditional braces, Six Month Smiles uses brackets and wires, but the brackets are clear and the wires are tooth-colored so as to be more discreet. Unlike traditional braces, Six Month Smiles only moves the teeth in the front of your smile. This is why you could have a new smile in six months (give or take a month or two).

Stains on your teeth naturally happen as you get older. The alignment of your teeth may be inherited from your parents. Even if you aren't affected by those issues, life happens, too. A game of catch with your nephew could end abruptly if one of you "catches" the ball with your mouth instead of your glove. A movie night with your family could end abruptly if someone bites into an unpopped kernel of popcorn.

For minor cracks or breaks, you may be able to restore the appearance of your tooth with **dental bonding**. For a deeper break, you may prefer a single dental veneer. And if the crack or break has damaged a large tooth, I can repair your smile with a dental crown.

The restorations I discussed previously can improve your appearance, too. Losing teeth can affect the shape of your face. By replacing missing teeth, you will be providing support for your facial muscles. Plus, you can have a smile that looks complete and natural once again, whether you need a crown, a bridge, or dentures.

Why People Get Cosmetic Dentistry

The decision to undergo a cosmetic dental treatment is a personal one. As one patient related to me, her granddaughter asked her one day why she didn't smile or kiss her and why she mumbled when she spoke.

This woman had been so concerned about hiding her teeth that she didn't realize how it had been affecting the people around her, the people she loved. Without that comment from her grandchild, she might still be living with the same issues that had bothered her for a long, long time.

In my experience, people are more likely to do something about their smiles when they have an emotional reason to do so.

I can't tell you how many patients have told me that they hated their smiles for years — even decades — before something convinced them that they needed to make a change. Some people are motivated to act because of a pending major life event, such as a wedding. This also can be the impetus they need to overcome their dental anxiety and improve their smiles.

For other people, an offhand comment from someone they've known for years, someone they love, or a stranger might convince them that hiding their smile is making a negative impression on other people.

I don't want you to live another day with a smile that leaves you feeling sad. I want you to live your life to the fullest, and I know based on what I've witnessed that a nice smile can help you be yourself. You don't have to wait until you get engaged and set the date for your wedding. You don't have to wait for your next high school or college reunion. You don't have to wait for a loved one to ask why you don't smile anymore.

If your fear of the dentist is preventing you from doing something you know you *want* to do, something you know you *should* do, then remember these two things.

First, no one at my practice will judge you because of the condition of your smile. Everyone at our office wants you to feel good about your teeth and about yourself. We're always happy to meet you where you are in your smile journey. We will be just as happy to help you get where you want to be.

Second, you can get any treatment you need for the smile you want without any pain. We have advanced technology, comfort options, and dental sedation for that very reason.

Patient Perspective: Art V.

Art used to become very self-conscious whenever someone took

38

out a camera or wanted to take his picture.

"My smiles were all with my lips closed. You know that kind of thing," he said.

It also affected his everyday interactions with people. During meetings at work, he felt very conscientious about where he sat.

"Everybody has their good side, their bad side, so you try to sit so this gap over here isn't the most pronounced part that people are going to see," Art said.

But his feelings about his teeth also made him apprehensive about getting help for his smile.

"One of the things that had kept me from seeing a dentist so long was the fear of the judgment: How did I get to this place, and how did I let this happen to my mouth and my teeth?" Art said.

After coming to our office, he has a new smile, and a new perspective on his life.

"I don't think about it anymore," Art said. "You know, I was always aware of it ... My teeth and the way I looked was always something I was concerned about and had to think about it. When I was eating, I had to think about, What am I going to eat and how am I going to eat?

"It's just a big weight that's gone."

Smile-Vision Before and After Photos

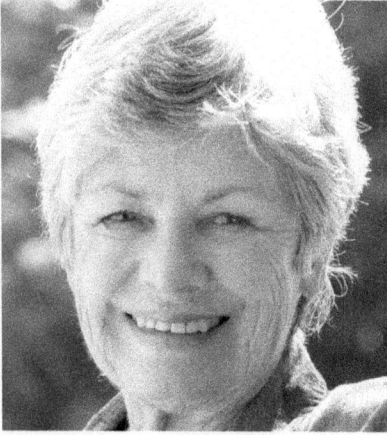

Before

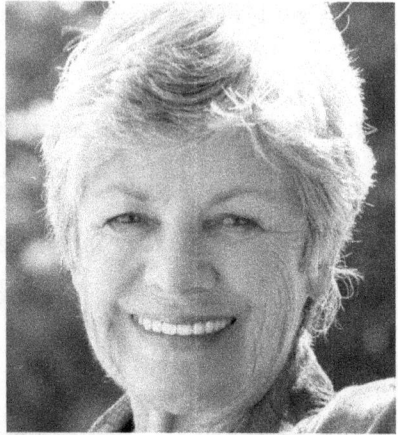

After

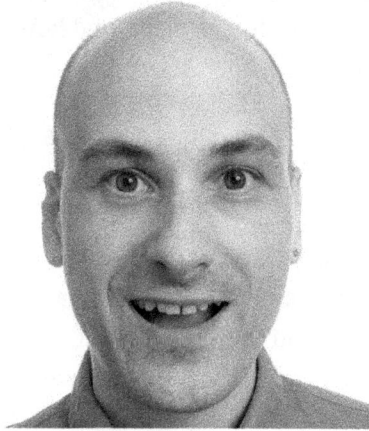

Before

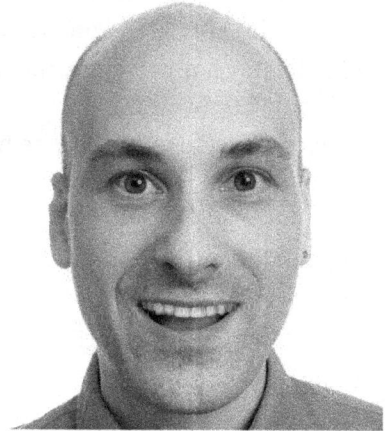

After

Comfort Menu

Newman Springs
Dental Care.com

Comfort Menu

- ☐ iPad
- ☐ TV with Headphones
- ☐ Magazine
- ☐ Crayons & Paper
- ☐ Blanket
- ☐ Nail Polish for Kids
- ☐ Chapstick
- ☐ Bottled Water
- ☐ Balloon Animal
- ☐ Sunglasses
- ☐ Neck Pillow
- ☐ Warm Towel
- ☐ Numbing Rinse

Feel free to pick any of our *Comfort Menu* choices.

7

How to Achieve Optimal Oral Health

Keeping your mouth as healthy as possible is a team effort.

You can keep your mouth healthy, but trying to do everything on your own is not the best approach. We can be your team. We can work with you to keep your smile looking great.

Of course, you do need to keep brushing *and* flossing every day. That will help you keep things from getting out of hand between your regular visits with us. Your routine checkups are when we may find problems that need more than a toothbrush and floss to fix. This also is when we can prevent problems you may not see by looking in the mirror each morning.

Getting to Know Us

Do you remember your first date with your spouse or significant other? You can probably recall being filled with excitement. You probably felt anxious, wondering if the person you were going out with would be someone you would like and trust. As you spent more time together, you felt more comfortable, less anxious, and even eager for the next time you would see him or her again.

Choosing a dentist may not be as romantic as finding the love of your life, but it is similar in some ways. If it's been a few years since your last dental visit, it can be nerve-wracking to make that first contact, whether by phone or online. I understand this. It's why I welcome you to stop by our office to meet me and my team *before* you schedule any treatment.

I want to start a conversation with you. This consultation is your opportunity to ask questions about me, about my approach to patient care, and about any of the services we offer, including sedation dentistry. This is your opportunity to tell me about your goals for your smile, whether you simply want to stay cavity-free or you want to have a smile that movie stars would envy.

I can explain how you can achieve your goals. I can even give you a map of how to get there. If you are ready for an appointment after getting to know more about me, my team, and what we can do for you, we'll be happy to reserve one for you.

Building a relationship with dental professionals you trust is important for maintaining your healthy smile.

As many people who fear the dentist have told me, a bad experience from their childhood often played a role in their feelings. Even if you are anxious about dental care, you don't want to pass those feelings on to your children. It's why we don't force children to have any treatment. If your son or daughter isn't ready for a cleaning just yet, we will wait until the next visit and try again.

Just like we do for our adult patients, we want to build good relationships with the kids who visit us. We want them to see the dentist office as a place where people want them to be happy and healthy.

Your Oral Health Affects Your Overall Health

A big part of why I became a dentist is that I wanted to help people. I'm also quite aware that your oral health affects your general health. This only makes me more motivated to encourage you and all my patients to keep making regular visits with my team and me.

Pain in your mouth is a clue that something is wrong with your teeth or gums. However, pain is often one of the last symptoms to develop. By the time you feel a toothache or sore gums, you already may have a fairly advanced problem.

As an example of what I mean, I had a patient at my office with a large hole in one tooth. It was so large that food was getting stuck in that tooth. I knew that a root canal would be the best way to take care of him and to restore his smile. He replied that his tooth didn't hurt, and he didn't think it was a real problem until we showed him a picture of it. At that point, he knew he had a choice to make. Either he could do something now and avoid the pain of a toothache, or he could wait until he was in serious pain and his tooth might need to be removed.

Oral infections have been linked to everything from cardiovascular disease to premature and low birthweight babies. If the bacteria in your mouth get into your bloodstream, they can contribute to infections and inflammation throughout your body. Periodontitis, an advanced form of gum disease, has been linked to heart disease and strokes. It's more common for people with diabetes to have gum disease, and gum disease can make it more difficult for diabetics to control their blood sugar levels. Researchers have found links between periodontal disease and osteoporosis, respiratory diseases, and an increased risk for some kinds of cancer, as well.

We routinely perform oral cancer screenings for our patients. The specialized light of our VELscope allows us to see differences in cell layers in your mouth and reveals unhealthy tissue. Early detection makes a world of difference in oral cancer treatment.

Losing your teeth can affect more than just your smile. When you are missing teeth, you aren't able to eat as many foods, and even with traditional dentures, you may not be able to chew your food as well as you should. This can lead to malnutrition, which could explain the studies showing that people with teeth live an average of 10 years longer than people without teeth. A healthy mouth is good for your well-being.

Admittedly, your oral health is not the only factor that can affect your overall health. Nevertheless, keeping your mouth as healthy as possible isn't going to hurt you, either.

Don't Grind Away Your Smile

When most people think about coming to the dentist, they think about preventing tooth decay or fixing cavities. These are excellent reasons to schedule dental appointments, but preventive care just scratches the surface of the things we can do to help you.

Millions of Americans grind or clench their teeth. The technical term for this is bruxism, and it can be incredibly disruptive in people's lives. Eight percent of the population grinds their teeth in their sleep, according to the National Sleep Foundation. That's 2 out of every 25 people.

This kind of grinding and clenching can wear down your tooth enamel and weaken your teeth, leaving them more vulnerable to bacteria, cavities, and tooth infections.

Teeth grinding can strain your jaw and facial muscles. An average adult is capable of biting with between 200 and 250 pounds of force. That's more than you need to eat pretty much anything, so it's rare for people to exert that much force in their everyday lives. In comparison, researchers have found that people who clench and grind their teeth can generate 500 pounds of pressure or more.

Imagine doing that for hours at a time every night while you sleep. That could explain frequent headaches, earaches, and jaw soreness. If you have these symptoms in the morning, that could be a clue that you are grinding your teeth in your sleep.

Why do people grind their teeth? It's possible that you have an alignment issue with your bite. You may have an injury as a result of trauma to your face or jaw. Arthritis or an illness could be affecting your jaw joint or the surrounding muscles.

Stress is another common reason people grind their teeth. Everyone can agree that life can be maddening at times. Work can be stressful. Family can be stressful, and financial matters can be stressful, too.

I may not be able to take away the stress in your life, but I may be able to save your teeth by creating a nightguard for you. You'll wear this custom-fitted oral appliance while you sleep.

The nightguard acts as a barrier between your upper and lower teeth, so you can't grind them together. The **nightguard** can help alleviate some symptoms of teeth grinding such as headaches and jaw pain, too. The reason is that the appliance can train your jaw to rest in a more relaxed position, reducing the strain on your jaw joint and the nearby muscle tissue.

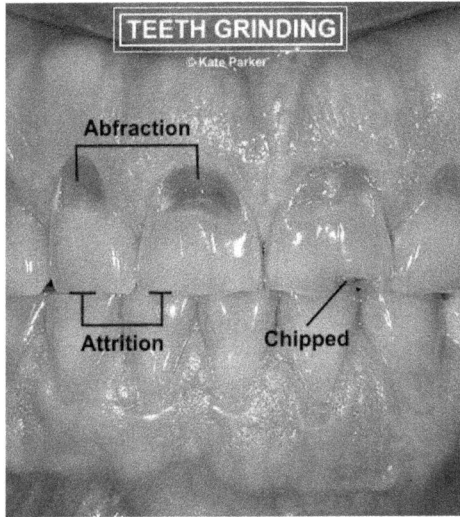

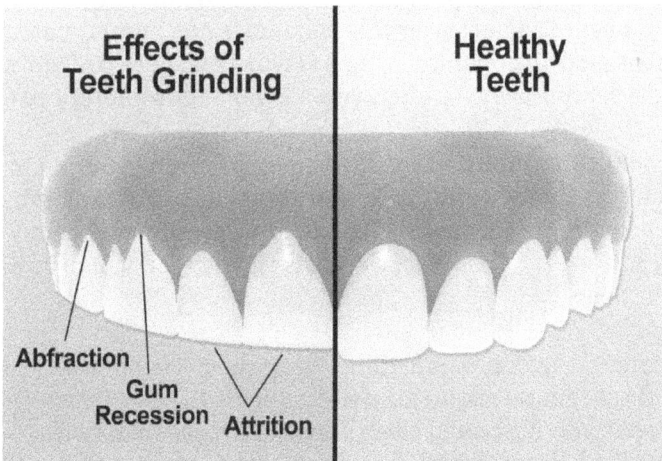

Stop Snoring & Sleep Better

Do you often wake up feeling like you hardly slept at all? Do people complain about your snoring? Do you catch yourself falling asleep when you are watching television, at your desk, or while you are driving?

Those signs could be the result of untreated sleep apnea, a sleep disorder in which people stop breathing when they fall asleep. The most common form is obstructive sleep apnea. Loud, constant snoring is one of its most noticeable symptoms.

This snoring can be so bad that people who sleep in the same bed, in the same room, or even in the same hallway can have *their* sleep interrupted. Snoring does not necessarily mean you have obstructive sleep apnea, but it is a clue that you should get tested.

According to the American Sleep Apnea Association, an estimated 22 million Americans have this condition, although most of them are not aware of it. Sleep apnea is not just a nuisance to other people when they are trying to sleep. It's keeping you from getting healthy sleep, and it's bad for your overall health.

You need deep, healthy sleep. When you have sleep apnea, you rarely stay asleep long enough to reach the stages of deep sleep. When you have obstructive sleep apnea, your airway will gradually close as you fade into sleep. The narrower this opening is, the more it vibrates the soft tissues near the opening, which is why you snore. You do stop snoring — temporarily — **when you airway is completely cut off**.

At that point, your brain will wake you up briefly so you can breathe again. Most of the time, this is so short that you won't remember it, although you may find yourself waking up occasionally feeling like you are gasping for air. The cycle starts again when you drift back into light sleep.

You become sleep deprived without deep sleep. People who are sleep deprived are more likely to fall asleep during the day, which could be why people with untreated sleep apnea are more than twice as likely to be involved in car accidents than other drivers.

Driving while drowsy is not the only risk of untreated sleep apnea. People with obstructive sleep apnea also have an increased risk of:

- Cardiovascular disease
- Diabetes
- Heart disease
- High blood pressure
- Stroke

So why am I taking time to discuss a sleep disorder? Believe it or not, a general dentist like me with the proper training can help you treat sleep apnea. I would be happy to talk to you if you or someone you care about might have obstructive sleep apnea. If you have already been diagnosed with sleep apnea but are having trouble with your CPAP machine, I can help you, too.

CPAP, or continuous positive airway pressure, has been the default treatment for sleep apnea for a long time. For a CPAP to work, you must wear a mask so the machine can push air through your mouth or nose into your airway. The air pressure forces your airway to stay open so you can continue breathing when you fall asleep. You stay asleep longer and get the healthy, deep sleep you need.

Unfortunately, many patients cannot adjust to sleeping with a mask on their face, or they find the mask irritating. Some people say the air pressure or the sound of the machine keeps them from falling asleep. Other people find that they remove their mask in their sleep. None of these patients is benefiting from CPAP treatment.

The FDA recently approved oral appliances to treat snoring and sleep apnea. The American Academy of Sleep Medicine also concluded that oral appliances can be a first-line treatment for people with mild or moderate sleep apnea and an alternate treatment for patients with severe sleep apnea who cannot tolerate a CPAP.

Like the nightguard for teeth grinding, this is a type of mouthguard. I can design a custom-fitted oral appliance for you or your loved one to wear while sleeping. These appliances work by slightly adjusting the position of your jaw to help your airway remain open. This reduces the volume and frequency of snoring. More importantly, it lets you keep breathing so you can enjoy deep, healthy sleep.

Could You Have Sleep Apnea?

Earlier I pointed out that most people with sleep apnea are not aware that they have it. If you don't know you have a problem, you probably aren't doing anything to fix it. For your sake or the sake of someone you love, please, take a moment to ask yourself a few questions.

- Do you often fall asleep while reading or watching television?
- Are you likely to doze off when you are seated in the same place for an extended time? This could be at your desk at work, in a car as a passenger, or in a movie theater.
- Are you likely to doze off if you lie down to rest in the afternoon?
- Do you often find that you are tired after eating lunch (without consuming any alcohol)?
- Have you ever dozed off while behind the wheel of a car?

I strongly encourage you to schedule a consultation with me soon if you said yes to more than one of these questions. You may not have sleep apnea, but it's not something you want to ignore if you do.

A Personal Concern

As a 22-year-old dental student, I started having neck pains. I was poring over books and studying hard, but that wasn't the cause of my problem. I was diagnosed with myofacial pain dysfunction. At the time, I was surprised to learn how much damage I had done to my teeth as a result of grinding.

Since then, I've worn a number of oral appliances to protect my teeth while I sleep. I started wearing a new kind of appliance about 10 years ago after I was diagnosed with mild sleep apnea. This appliance still protects my teeth from the damage of clenching and grinding, but it has also allowed me to get deep, healthy sleep.

I'm sharing this because I want you to know that I take a special interest whenever I see a patient who shows symptoms of bruxism or sleep apnea. I know how both conditions can affect your life. I've lived with both problems, which is why it's so important to me to help you.

To Your Healthy Smile

You will always be welcome at Newman Springs Dental Care, no matter how long it's been since your last dental visit. We are happy to meet new patients and welcome them into our dental family.

Your comfort and your health are interconnected. We want you to feel at ease so you can get the care you need and deserve. We go above and beyond the basics of keeping you free from cavities and gum disease. We want to protect your smile, help you get quality sleep, and improve your quality of life.

Patient Perspective: Jack F.

Jack admits that he was a quite surprised when he first visited my office.

"Usually, the dentist is very either standoffish, or they're very quick to take a look at something and get it done and get you out. Here, I felt very comfortable about the way it was handled and the customer service end of it," he said.

Jack added that he felt his initial exam was complete and thorough, but that's not the only reason he came back.

"It was done in an atmosphere that didn't make me feel like I had to go get dental work done right away or I was in terror," he said.

From the start until the end of his treatment, we provided Jack with professional and comfortable service.

"I was very hesitant to come to a dentist, as most people are, but I think after one or two visits here and some of the work that was done, seeing what happened to me, I felt very good about it," he said. "I think that I'd recommend it to anyone. Give it a try."

8

When You Are Ready, I'll Be Here to Help

Keeping your mouth healthy takes more than just finding a good dentist. You need to find a dentist you trust.

Dentistry isn't like fixing a computer. It involves more than just making mechanical changes to repair, replace, improve, and maintain your smile. To get the best dental care, you need to find someone you feel comfortable talking to about your worries and your goals.

When I realized how much dental anxiety and fear of the dentist was preventing people from getting care they needed and deserved, I sought training in dental sedation. I didn't stop until I met the requirements to offer three types of sedation dentistry.

My goal has always been to help anyone who visits my family practice. We are happy to care for patients from 2 years old to 102 years old. My sedation training gave me the tools to help more people than ever. Today, one of the best parts of my job is seeing patients become less anxious about dental care and more comfortable with their smiles.

What I Will Do for You

From the first moment you call my office, walk through the door, or sit in one of my chairs, I want you to be untroubled. My team and I want to get to know *you*, not just your oral health condition. We want to understand why you may feel apprehensive about dental care. That's also why we want to answer your questions so you can feel at ease.

Your comfort is one of our highest priorities. As I explained in chapter 2, it fits perfectly with our core values. Our guests' needs always come first at Newman Springs Dental Care. We strive to be warm, caring, enthusiastic, and lighthearted. We want you to feel like you are part of our family any time you visit us.

Whether you want to restore, enhance, or maintain your smile, I am confident that I have the training, experience, tools, and team to turn the smile of your dreams into the smile you see in your reflection.

I'll Be Here for You

Regardless of how bad you think your oral health may be, I am here to support you. We offer free, friendly phone advice, and we are always happy to help.

No matter how fearful you may be about coming to the dentist, our team wants you to feel comfortable and comforted. Your emotional well-being is as important to us as your dental health.

Please contact me when you are ready to make an appointment or if you just want to learn more about my approach to dentistry. I hope to hear from you soon, and I look forward to meeting you in person again or for the first time.

Newman Springs
Dental Care.com

539 Newman Springs Road
Lincroft, NJ 07738
732-352-3903
www.BestLincroftDentist.com

About the Author

Dr. Mitchel Friedman was one of the first dentists licensed to offer dental sedation by the New Jersey State Board of Dentistry. He remains one of the few general dentists in New Jersey with the training to offer three forms of sedation — nitrous oxide, oral sedation, and IV sedation — in his office.

Dr. Friedman has been practicing dentistry since 1984 in Monmouth County, NJ, where he was born and raised. He graduated from Middletown Township High School in 1976, then completed his bachelor's degree at Rutgers College. He earned his Doctor of Dental Surgery from the Medical College of Virginia School of Dentistry, where he graduated in the top 15 percent of his class.

He returned to his home community, where he completed an advanced general dental residency at Monmouth Medical Center before going into private practice. He has completed more than 1,500 hours of continuing education and received his Mastership in the Academy of General Dentistry, a distinction only 2 percent of dentists have earned. He also serves as a part-time clinical instructor at Monmouth Medical Center, where he teaches advanced techniques and sedation to recent dental graduates.

Outside the office, Dr. Friedman enjoys working on his classic cars (a

1972 MGB and a 1960 MGA) and doing home repairs. He also enjoys boating, fishing, scuba diving, skiing, and tennis. His wife, Adrienne, is a chemistry teacher. They have three adult children: Gillian, Jared, and Hannah.

.

www.ingramcontent.com/pod-product-compliance
Lightning Source LLC
Chambersburg PA
CBHW070945210326
41520CB00021B/7067